Marina Zimmermann

Effect of cryoprotectant dilution on equine semen

Marina Zimmermann

Effect of cryoprotectant dilution on equine semen

Evaluation of in vitro sperm motility and viability parameters in the dilution of the cryoprotectant dimethylformamide

ScienciaScripts

Imprint
Any brand names and product names mentioned in this book are subject to trademark, brand or patent protection and are trademarks or registered trademarks of their respective holders. The use of brand names, product names, common names, trade names, product descriptions etc. even without a particular marking in this work is in no way to be construed to mean that such names may be regarded as unrestricted in respect of trademark and brand protection legislation and could thus be used by anyone.

Cover image: www.ingimage.com

This book is a translation from the original published under ISBN 978-613-9-68895-1.

Publisher:
Sciencia Scripts
is a trademark of
Dodo Books Indian Ocean Ltd. and OmniScriptum S.R.L publishing group

120 High Road, East Finchley, London, N2 9ED, United Kingdom
Str. Armeneasca 28/1, office 1, Chisinau MD-2012, Republic of Moldova, Europe
Printed at: see last page
ISBN: 978-620-8-24084-4

CONTENTS

DEDICATORY

I dedicate this to my dear mother for completing yet another stage; for her strength and support in carrying out the postgraduate course, as well as the experiments; for her values, education, culture, interest in everything around us, for her conversations, scolding, trust, love, affection, dedication and for "putting my feet on the ground".

I would also like to dedicate it to my father, *in memoriam*, for his respect, affection, love, childhood letters, sweet "beatings", joy, sensitivity, humanity, protection and for "getting my feet off the ground".

Finally, I dedicate it to my dear cousin *Don Juan*, for the strength, joy, friendliness, charm and message of life that he left us.

ACKNOWLEDGMENTS

To Professor Dr. Jairo Pereira Neves for his guidance, trust, teachings, conversations and discussions.

To my large and loving family for their understanding, help, education and culture.

To the dear friends I made during this course, especially my colleague Juliana Lopes Almeida, and to those who have followed my journey.

To Professor Jûlio Jacob, Vera Jesus and José Eugênio Três at UFRRJ for the first lessons in Animal Reproduction, trust, encouragement and friendship.

To Professor Dr. Frederico Ozanam Papa of UNESP/Campus Botucatu - SP for the use of his laboratory, his teachings and his dedication, as well as to his advisors Ms. Cely Marini Melo and Dr. José A. Dell'Aqua Jr. for their promptness and availability of time.

To Dr. Rodolfo Rumpf, Dr. Roberto Sartori and Dr. Margot N. Dode of EMBRAPA/CENARGEN - DF for making the laboratory available for semen processing, as well as making the animals available.

To the Veterinary Doctor Adalberto Farinasso for his ideas and trust.

To Professor Dr. Clàudio Del Menezzi for his help with the review and statistical calculations.

Especially to my uncles Clóvis and Sinhô and cousins André and Luiz Gustavo, for the loan of materials and animals to carry out the experiment.

To the staff, Japao, Teco, Cowboy and Pelé for their help and patience.

To the professors of the postgraduate course in Agricultural Sciences at FAV/UnB.

To the National Council for Scientific and Technological Development - CNPq, for the financial support.

SUMMARY:

The aim of this study was to evaluate *in vitro* motility and viability parameters when diluting the 5% post-thaw cryoprotectant dimethylformamide to concentrations of 2.5 and 1.25%, using two commercial diluents added to cryopreserved equine semen. After thawing, the samples were diluted in order to maintain the final concentrations (2.5 and 1.25%) of cryoprotectant, using two commercial diluents (FR4® and Botu-Crio®) at two times: initial (Ti) and final (Tf). Thirteen different ejaculate samples from five national breed sires were used. Motility parameters were observed using computerized analysis and plasma membrane integrity using epifluorescence microscopy. There was an improvement in the total and progressive motility parameters of the spermatozoa at the final time ($P<0.05$) with the Botu-Crio diluent® compared to FR4® . There was no difference, $P > 0.05$, between the treatments in terms of plasma membrane integrity.

Keywords: equine, diluent , cryoprotectant , freezing, thawing

1 INTRODUCTION

Once the commercial interest in the use of artificial insemination (AI) with frozen semen became apparent, research into the cryopreservation of equine semen has been constantly implemented and developed, although the results are still unsatisfactory in terms of fertility rates.

In addition to genetic improvement, the freezing of semen serves as a genetic reserve bank for animals of high racial and commercial standard, promotes greater exchange between breeders from various regions and countries and selects individuals and strains in terms of their fertility and freezability. Cryopreservation helps to minimize economic losses resulting from the death of breeding stock of high commercial value or which take part in breed revitalization programs, to preserve native breeds from extinction and to conserve endangered species, and also to overcome aspects of male infertility in humans (WATSON, 2000).

The cryopreservation of equine semen, as well as that of several other species, has not yet reached a standardized technique that provides satisfactory and repeatable results, as is the case with the bovine species (WATSON, 2000). Most research is carried out to improve the cryopreservation technique, with a view to obtaining more consistent results. There was no selection of sires in terms of fertility or even freezability, which favored the permanence of a large number of sires with low fertility.

The use of cryoprotective agents in the semen freezing process is necessary to maintain the viability of sperm cells, as they protect these cells from damage caused by thermal shock, due to the formation of ice crystals, dehydration and subsequent thawing (SNOECK, 2002). However, these agents also cause deleterious toxic effects to sperm cells when added to or removed from them (BALL & VOSS, 2001).

The aim of this study was to evaluate *in vitro* the effects of diluting the post-thaw cryoprotectant to concentrations of 2.5 and 1.25% using two commercial diluents on equine semen cryopreserved with diluent containing the cryoprotectant dimethylformamide at 5%.

2. BACKGROUND

Over the past decade, we have witnessed an explosion of biotechnological advances in the field of animal breeding. Some of these technologies have been routinely incorporated into the "horse industry", others are being incorporated more slowly or some never will be. The rate at which these technologies are accepted and used in the equine breeding industry depends on their success, the attitude and work of professionals in the field and, above all, the cost/benefit ratio. The number of mares inseminated with frozen semen has been increasing, particularly in the USA, which has boosted studies related to semen freezing and attracted greater investment to the area (SQUIRES, 2005).

Since the last decade, some horse breeders' associations, such as those for the Arabian horse, the Quarter Horse, the American Paint Horse, the Brazilian Equestrian, among others, have allowed the use of frozen semen. As of this year, the Mangalarga Marchador and Campolina horse associations have decided to allow the use of the technique, opening up the national market for frozen equine semen.

The biggest limitation to the use of frozen semen in the equine species stems from the great individual variability in sperm freezability due to genetic and environmental factors. Most stallions have peculiar post-thaw semen characteristics (sperm motility and cell membrane integrity) that are unsuitable for use (SQUIRES *et al.*, 1999), and there is even a specific common name: "bad freezers" and "good freezers", for animals that freeze badly and well, respectively. Semen from good freezer stallions provides average post-thaw progressive sperm motility between 40-70% and fertility rates between 60-75% per cycle, in mares inseminated with 300×10^6 spermatozoa, 24 hours before and six hours after ovulation. In the case of poorly frozen stallions, this figure drops to less than 30% conception rate per cycle (CRISTIANELLI et al., 1984; HAARD & HAARD, 1991; JASKO et al., 1992; THOMASSEN, 1993; BOYLE, 1999).

Many studies have focused on identifying the damage caused to sperm during the freezing and thawing process. There appear to be two major classes of sperm damage: oxidative and osmotic.

SQUIRES (2005), concluded that most of the progress in increasing the survival of frozen and thawed spermatozoa is focused on minimizing oxidative stress and decreasing osmotic stress. One of the factors that may be involved in the variability of the post-thaw response of equine semen is the use of glycerol as a cryoprotective agent (DEMICK et al., 1976).

The higher the fertility rates using simpler AI protocols, the greater the credibility of the technique and its use will certainly become more constant. With this, the routine of inseminations with frozen semen in equine breeding centres and even in stud farms is likely to increase, minimizing losses with semen transport (currently done with cooled semen), reducing the number of collections from stallions that are overused for semen sales (which brings numerous benefits from the animal's welfare point of view) and certainly genetic gain.

According to WATSON (2000), the process of cryopreserving semen results in a decrease in fertility when compared to fresh semen and for this reason, the search to increase the fertility rate should not only be focused on freezing protocols, but also on protocols that allow for greater functional ability of the sperm population that has survived the entire freezing/thawing process.

3. LITERATURE REVIEW

3.1 Composition of the piasmatic membrane

According to FLESCH & GADELLA (2000), although there is considerable variation between different species of mammals, the plasma membrane is made up of approximately 70% phospholipids (phosphocholine glyceride - PC, phosphoethanolamine glyceride - PE, phosphatidylserine - PS, phosphatidylinositol - PI and cardiolipin - CL), 25% neutral lipids (cholesterol - the most variable factor between ejaculates from the same individual and between individuals and species - desmosterol, cholesterol sulphate and cholesterol esters) and 5% glycolipids (seminolipids).

Differences in the amount of cholesterol in the piasmatic membrane may not only be related to capacitation indices, but may also affect fertility and the ability of a stallion's ejaculate to withstand cooling and freezing (YANAGUIMACHI et al., 1994). MINELLI et al. (1998) reported that seminal plasma can block the efflux of cholesterol from the piasmatic membrane via prostasomes, which are cholesterol-rich prostatic vesicles. The fluidity of the membrane depends on the temperature, its cholesterol content and its lipid composition, with the length and degree of unsaturation of the fatty acid chains being important.

Of interest to andrologists is the fact that cooling semen for freezing can lead to phase transitions, as well as protein bundles (DE LEEUW, 1990). The transition phase is due to a re-organization of the hydrocarbon chains, which move from a fluid and disordered state to a gel state, which is the one with the most pronounced organization. This phase occurs as a result of changes in temperature (STR YER, 1992). For the equine sperm cell, the transition phase occurs at a temperature of 20.7°C (AMMAN & GRAHAM, 1993).

Studies on human semen freezing have concluded that membrane fluidity decreases after cryopreservation and that resistance to freezing and thawing processes is better in individuals with high membrane fluidity. The variation in this fluidity may explain the variability in sperm freezing, a fact that is observed between individual sires (GIRAUD et al., 2000).

Due to the large amount of unsaturated fatty acids in the plasma membrane, mammalian spermatozoa are highly sensitive to oxidative stress. Semen processing involves numerous factors that cause damage to the plasma membrane of spermatozoa including semen collection, the addition of semen diluents, centrifugation, cooling, freezing and thawing (AURICH, 2005).

When compared to other species, such as sheep, the plasma membrane of equine spermatozoa has a higher cholesterol content, estimated at 37%. However, this content differs not only between species, but also between individuals of the same species and even between ejaculates from the same individual (GADELLA et al., 2001).

3.2 Sperm capacity

It is quite possible that the time required to optimize sperm capacitation is related to the slow efflux of cholesterol from unresponsive sub-populations of sperm cells. This idea is supported by the fact that species with large amounts of cholesterol, such as humans and cattle, require longer periods for optimal capacitation (six and eight hours respectively), while wild boar and sheep, which have a small amount of cholesterol content, only need one or two hours for capacitation (YANAGUIMACHI et al., 1994).

Prostasomes (cholesterol-rich vesicles secreted by the prostate) are found in the seminal plasma of humans and stallions. These prostasomes block the efflux of cholesterol from sperm cells and probably serve to delay capacitation (CROSS, 1998).

Physiological changes in the plasma membrane after ejaculation are essential for the capacitation process and are associated with the activation of the fertilizing capacity of sperm cells and also lead to a different model of motility called hypermotility (YANAGUIMACHI et al., 1994).

Damage to the plasma membrane of spermatozoa results in irreversible loss of motility and/or fertilization capacity. During ejaculation and in the female genital tract, spermatozoa are subjected to numerous factors that can damage their plasma membrane or induce cell death. This is why only hundreds to thousands of cells, out of the billions that were ejaculated, will reach the oviduct

(MORRIS et al., 2000).

3.3 Freezability

During the cooling and freezing of semen, sperm undergo a series of physical and chemical changes which include: partial dehydration, penetration of cryoprotectants into the cell, structural reorganization of membrane lipids and proteins, exposure to high solute concentrations and inter- and intracellular exposure to ice crystals (HENRY et al., 2002; SNOECK, 2002). Cryopreservation protocols are designed to minimize these negative effects of stress.

According to PICKETT (1986), cell damage is caused by the formation of intracellular ice crystals that affect the structure of the cell, by the concentration of the solute resulting from the freezing of pure water and by the interaction between these two factors. In equine sperm, these factors are minimized by controlling the cooling rate between critical temperatures (19°C and 8°C) and by adding a diluent containing lipids such as egg yolk or lipoproteins such as milk. The freezing point of the cell cytoplasm is normally below -1°C, with cells generally remaining unfrozen in the -10°C to -15°C range, i.e. they are cool even in the presence of ice. This indicates that the plasma membrane can prevent the spread of extracellular ice into the supercooled cell (ZÙCCARI, 1998).

In thawing, the cells are exposed to the same factors, but in the opposite way: cell rehydration by the entry of water into the cell through the plasma membrane to balance the osmolarity, which is created when the extracellular crystals are melted. The lipids and proteins of the plasma membrane are reorganized and the cryoprotectant is diffused out of the cells (PICKETT, 1986). Sperm are sensitive to many environmental factors, including temperature, light, physical damage and other chemicals. Shock or even small variations in temperature cause disruption of the structural lipids in the plasma membrane and thus damage to the spermatozoa (PICKETT, 1992).

Há great loss in the viability of sperm cells after thawing and sublethal dysfunction in a proportion of the surviving subpopulation. The losses incurred in the cryopreservation process are compensated for by the insemination of a large number of spermatozoa, and this is true both for bull semen and for other species (WATSON, 2000). It is estimated that only 30-40% of sires produce semen of good quality for the freezing process, and a consistent variation in sperm freezability is observed between species (ALVARENGA et al., 2003).

Many characteristics of spermatozoa are considered important for fertilization and must be maintained after cryopreservation when good fertilization capacity is expected: progressive motility, normal metabolism, intact cell membrane, presence of acrosomal enzymes, intact surface proteins responsible for sperm-ovocyte interaction and uninjured nucleoproteins. Cryopreserved sperm undergo various stresses associated with the freezing, thawing and insemination process, which can make them non-viable. Most damage to spermatozoa results from structural changes in the plasma membrane, osmotic shock, dehydration, the formation of intracellular ice crystals, fluctuations in cell volume/surface area or metabolic imbalances (BLANCHARD et al., 2003).

3.4 Thinners

As a way of optimizing semen quality and protecting it, extender media or diluents are added to the semen after collection. These are preheated to 37°C and mostly homogenized with the semen in a 1:1 ratio (BLANCHARD et al., 2003).

The osmotic pressure of the extenders should be between 300 and 400 mOsmol/L, with 350 mOsmol/L being optimal, and the pH between 6.7 and 7.2, with 6.7 and 6.9 being considered ideal. These factors contribute to maximizing sperm survival and linear motility (BLANCHARD et al., 2003). In other words, the appropriate diluent must have an osmotic pressure compatible with that of the spermatozoa, a pH similar to that of the semen (which is between 6.7 and 7.2) balanced with mineral elements and also have substances capable of neutralizing toxic products (antibiotics) and providing protection against thermal shock (AMANN & PICKETT, 1987; BRINSKO & VARNER, 1998). It is also known that the osmolarity of seminal fluid is approximately 300 mOsmol/Kg (PICKETT et al., 1993).

Diluents based on milk or egg yolk are commonly used in horses. Most contain a source of lipoproteins, and milk proteins are capable of stabilizing protein elements in the sperm membrane (WATSON, 1981). HOCHACHKA (1986) observed that casein binds strongly to Ca^{++} ions, which prevents the intracellular accumulation of toxic amounts of Ca^{++} resulting from membrane damage. Lipoproteins are bound to the plasma membrane and promote its stabilization during the freezing/thawing process.

MELO et al. (2005) observed that there was no influence of the diluents used in centrifugation on the parameters analyzed for the freezing of equine semen, demonstrating that the different milk-based diluents are efficient in the centrifugation of ejaculates, in the freezing process and indicating the importance of carrying out individual freezability tests. Associations of cryoprotectants were compared prior to definitive freezing and this is a possible alternative for increasing the fertility of frozen semen in the equine species. In another study by MARTIN et al. (2005), it was observed that replacing whole egg yolk with 8% LDL in the diluent modified by MARTIN et al. (1979) proved to be beneficial for the viability of cryopreserved equine spermatozoa.

3.5 Toxicity of cryoprotectants to the piasmatic membrane

Glycerol is the most common cryoprotective agent used in equine semen freezing media (AMMAN & PICKET, 1987), although it greatly alters the selective permeability of the cell membrane to water and ions, and is toxic to spermatozoa at high concentrations, impairing fertility (GRAHAM, 1996).

HAMMERSTEDT and GRAHAM (1992) reported other effects caused by glycerol, which include: changes in cytoplasmic events such as increased viscosity due to intracellular glycerol, altered tubulin polymerization, changes in microtubule association, effects on the bioenergetic balance and direct changes in the plasma membrane and glycocalyx. This toxicity is due to osmotic stress, because glycerol is slower to enter the cell membrane than other cryoprotectants. Therefore, glycerol has a direct effect on the plasma membrane, altering its fluidity (GILMORE et al., 1995).

The toxic effects of glycerol can be osmotic in nature, due to changes in the organization, fluidity and permeability of the membrane, as well as biochemical injuries, which occur due to the interaction

between this cryoprotectant and the components of the spermatozoa (WATSON, 1995). BALL &
VOSS (2001) evaluated the osmotic tolerance of equine spermatozoa in relation to the addition and
removal of different agents, concluding that the addition and removal of glycerol resulted in greater
osmotic stress, characterized by a reduction in motility and a decrease in cellular and acrosomal
integrity, when compared to the other cryoprotectants studied.

3.6 Cryoprotectants

The first pregnancy in horses using semen cryopreserved with the cryoprotectant glycerol was
reported in 1957 (BARKER, 1957). In addition to glycerol, other substances such as ethylene glycol,
dimethyl sulfoxide (DMSO) and propylene glycol have been used successfully to freeze embryos and
have been evaluated for the cryopreservation of semen from other species (JEYENDRAN, 1980).

The variation in cell volume due to the entry and exit of the cryoprotectant and water (osmotic shock)
is believed to be one of the main causes of low semen viability after thawing. The use of
cryoprotectants with greater permeability to sperm cells is desirable due to the possibility of
minimizing osmotic shock (GOMES et al., 2002).

ASHWOOD-SMITH (1987) classified cryoprotectants into two groups: alcohols (ethylene glycol,
propylene glycol, glycerol) and amides. He suggested that the ideal cryoprotectant should have a low
molecular weight, good water solubility and minimal toxicity to sperm. As most amides have a lower
molecular weight than glycerol (glycerol has a molecular weight of 92, methyl formamide 59 and
dimethyl formamide 73), these cryoprotective agents should induce less osmotic damage as they
penetrate the sperm plasma membrane more quickly. The sensitivity of spermatozoa to the damaging
effects of glycerol is species-dependent. For species such as rabbits, chickens and fish, glycerol has
proved ineffective and amides have emerged as an alternative for freezing semen in these species.

Following WATSON (1995), DMSO seems to be a good cryoprotectant for rabbit and elephant
spermatozoa and in one study, it showed the best motility and viability values post-thawing and
increased the post-thawing results of sires that froze poorly when cryopreserved with glycerol. In

another experiment, CHENIER et al. (1998), reported that there was no significant difference in freezability between glycerol, ethylene glycol and DMSO when data from all sires were analyzed, although DMSO did improve post-thaw characteristics when compared to the other treatments. Compared to glycerol and DMSO, ethylene glycol was able to decrease the progressive post-thaw motility of equine spermatozoa. In the same study, semen frozen with diethylene glycol and propylene glycol showed lower post-thaw motility and viability than the other cryoprotective agents.

According to MELLO et al. (2005), the addition of the cryoprotectant in multiple stages, associated with cooling the sample slowly before the freezing process, is the most effective treatment for preserving the viability of equine sperm cells. Based on laboratory and field fertility evaluation methodologies, the combination of glycerol and dimethyl formamide has proved to be an alternative for cryopreserving equine sperm (NEVES NETO et al., 2004). In his study, SILVA (2005) used the cryoprotectant dimethyl formamide (DMF) alone or in association with glycerol and ethylene glycol and found the former to be more effective than the latter two in the cryopreservation of semen from Brazilian Pony breed horses. Interestingly, a study by OLIVEIRA et al. (2006) concluded that the cryoprotectants used in the experiment were effective in protecting sperm during the freezing and thawing process of semen from national breeds of donkeys. However, despite the good *in vitro* results, no pregnant animals were inseminated with the frozen semen.

3.7 Amides

Amides have been shown to be efficient for freezing in various animal species, including horses. The amides have shown very favorable results in the various sperm parameters evaluated, especially for stallions which show unfavorable results with the use of glycerol (ALVARENGA et al., 2000). In general, amides are less toxic to sperm when compared to glycerol (AMMAN & PICKET, 1987; GRAHAM, 1996). The efficiency of amides may be related to their lower molecular weight compared to glycerol, which provides greater permeability in the plasma and acrosomal membranes, consequently causing less osmotic damage to the spermatozoa (MEDEIROS et al., 2003).

Some experiments have shown that dimethyl formamide (DMF) preserved equine spermatozoa similarly to glycerol (ALVARENGA et al., 1996; KEITH, 1998), when used in sires with high freezability rates. According to ALVARENGA et al. (2005), the lower viscosity and lower molecular weight of amides favor greater permeability of these components within the plasma membrane.

VIDAMENT et al. (2002) found no improvement in the quality of equine semen cryopreserved using 1%, 3% and 5% glycerol with different concentrations of DMF (1% and 3%) when compared to the use of glycerol alone (GLY). In a similar experiment using the ejaculate of twenty stallions of different breeds, MEDEIROS et. al (2002) observed that semen frozen with DMF alone resulted in greater motility (p<0.05) than other cryoprotectants. The disagreement between the two authors can be explained by the fact that there were differences between the experiments due to the number and variability of the stallions used. In the first, only horses with good freezability were used; in the second, there was a greater variety of breeds and, as a result, great variability in the quality of the frozen semen used.

MEDEIROS et al. (2002) also showed that post-thaw motility (total and progressive) was higher when spermatozoa were frozen in the presence of 3% dimethyl acetamide (DMA) compared to 5% glycerol, although motility was similar in the presence of 5% DF or 5% methyl formamide (MF). The total and progressive motility results for the different treatments were: DMA 3% (50% and 15%); MF 5% (49% and 10%); DMF 5% (52% and 12%); and GLY 5% (27% and 8%).

In an experiment using 55 stallions of different breeds (Quarter Horse, Thoroughbred, Arabian, Campolina, Mangalarga Marchador and Lusitano), 5% DMF or 5% GLY was used as a cryoprotectant. Comparing the two, the results showed better total progressive motility in 40 of the 55 stallions when DMF was used; the percentage of progressive motility of the sperm frozen with GLY post-thawing was higher than 40% in 38% (21/55) and above 80% (44/55) for the group that used DMF. A comparison of the data from all the sires showed that DMF was superior (p<0.05) in maintaining total post-thaw motility (DMF=50% and GLY=33%) and progressive sperm motility (DMF=19% compared to GLY=15%) (ALVARENGA et al., 2003).

In another experiment with frozen semen using an extender containing lactose EDTA with DMF or

GLY, MOFFET et al. (2003) showed no improvement in motility, although pregnancy rates were higher in mares inseminated with the diluting medium containing DMF (47%, 14/30), compared to the group with medium containing GLY (14%, 5/34). Based on these data, they concluded that glycerol can reduce the fertility rates of frozen semen, even if sperm motility and viability are preserved.

In contrast, VIDAMENT et al. (2002) showed no differences in fertility rates in mares inseminated with semen that had been frozen with diluents containing DMF or GLY; the mares were inseminated daily and the pregnancy rates for those inseminated with frozen semen containing 2% GLY or 2% DMF were 46 and 50%, respectively.

In studies with rabbits, the use of dimethylformamide was shown to better preserve sperm motility after thawing when compared to glycerol (HANADA & NAGASE, 1980); however, WILMUT & POLGE (1977) observed that dimethylformamide promoted lower sperm motility after thawing semen from humans and sheep.

3.8 Laboratory evaluations

Many attempts to determine membrane integrity were based on the idea that an intact plasma membrane could prevent the death of sperm cells by preventing substances from the external environment from entering their cytoplasm. This was first studied using eosin or eosin combined with nigrosin stains (DOTT & FOSTER, 1972).

Routine evaluations or spermograms of fresh semen show: sperm motility, morphology, membrane integrity, the number of sperm per ejaculate and the volume and color of the ejaculate. However, these characteristics have not yet been significantly correlated with stallion fertility (NEILD et al., 1999; TORRES-BOGGINO et al., 1994), but they serve as a parameter as they are included in the standards established by the Brazilian College of Animal Reproduction - CBRA (1998) for equine sperm characteristics.

Currently, fluorescent stains, such as propidium iodide (PI), carboxyfluorescein acetate (CFDA) or

SYBR-14, are used successfully to evaluate equine semen (HARKEMA & BOYLE, 1992; HARRISON & VICKERS, 1990). Fluorescent dyes with an affinity for DNA are not permeable to intact cells, so only dead cells are stained red, while intact cells are stained green. Fluorescent probes include ethidium bromide, propidium iodide and hydroethidine, among others (ZÙCCARI, 1998). HARRISON & VICKERS (1990) added formaldehyde to the technique so that the cells would remain static without suffering structural damage. This method made it possible to evaluate wet preparations for epifluorescence microscopy, making it a more economically viable alternative to flow cytometry.

Most studies on the functional integrity of the plasma membrane still use sperm motility as their main marker. Despite the importance of membrane integrity for sperm motility, this depends on energy production from the mitochondrial compartment of the sperm midpiece (BRITO et al., 2003). The limitation of subjective evaluation of sperm motility by optical and phase contrast microscopy is being replaced by the use of computer assisted sperm analysis (CASA). There are different systems and manufacturers of CASA and it not only makes it possible to determine the percentage of motile and immotile spermatozoa, but also to characterize the motility pattern of the sperm cell in humans, bulls, stallions, dogs, sheep and laboratory animals (VERSTEGEN et al., 2002). Combinations of different velocity patterns allow the definition of different sperm subpopulations and tend to correlate better with fertility than a simple velocity parameter alone (ABAIGAR et al., 1999). The sperm analysis obtained through CASA allows the determination of various parameters for motility and the evaluation of morphological aberrations (THURSTON et al., 1999).

Thus, each computerized analysis system requires standardization in semen sample preparation, machine calibration and technical efficiency in order to obtain accurate and repeatable results (SCHÀFER-SOMI & AURICH, 2006). Some authors have drawn attention to CASA's ability to predict individual sire fertility, since its data must be correlated with *in vivo* fertility studies (VIZCARRA & FORD, 2006). According to VERSTEGEN et al. (2002), the biggest problem related to CASA is the standardization and optimization of the equipment and its procedures by its operators; although they report that all the different computerized analysis equipment has demonstrated high levels of accuracy and reliable results, as it is a great tool for providing objective comparisons of motility with sperm morphology.

However, for scientific research purposes, the computerized sperm analysis system has become a very valuable tool as it provides a reliable assessment of sperm movements.

3.9 Frozen semen and the uterine environment, implications

When the number of sperm or their quality in insemination is reduced, fertility declines in an exponential curve. Normally, insemination is done with a sufficient number of competent sperm to achieve the best results. If the total number of viable sperm in an insemination with frozen semen falls below the number needed for a good fertilization rate, then fertility will be reduced (HUNTER, 1984).

LOOMIS (2001) observed that the fertility of frozen semen in commercial programs ranged from 32 - 73% in mares inseminated only once to 56 - 89% in mares inseminated more than once during the breeding season, noting that the fertility of frozen semen is influenced by numerous factors, including: sperm quality, stallion selection, insemination dose, selection of the dam and management.

For insemination with frozen semen to be successful, as well as having good post-thawing standards, it is essential to have a reproductive history of the mares to be used, to carry out daily follicular monitoring and to use the best technique for depositing the semen in the uterine environment. Females over the age of eight with a history of reproductive problems generally have low pregnancy rates and are potential candidates for not conceiving (SAMPER et al., 2001). Persistent post-insemination endometritis, fluid accumulation or the occurrence of uterine edema can seriously reduce the chances of pregnancy in females (TROEDSSON et al., 1995). Post-insemination uterine inflammation or acute endometritis following the use of frozen semen is no more severe than with fresh or chilled semen, but appears to be more long-lasting (METCALF, 2000) and can vary according to the concentration of sperm deposited and the cryoprotective agent used.

According to KOTILAINEN et al. (1994) frozen semen does not induce greater uterine inflammation than fresh semen, but due to the reduced volume and high sperm concentration, the uterine response tends to be stronger than when other types of semen are used. The high proportion of dead spermatozoa when mares are inseminated with frozen semen suggests a reason for the high uterine inflammatory response; however, the dead spermatozoa did not induce a greater influx of polymorphonuclear cells into the uterine fluid than the live spermatozoa deposited in the uterus of mares inseminated with fresh semen (KATILA, 1997).

In one study, LOOMIS & SQUIRES (2005) observed the presence of post-insemination uterine fluid in 23% of mares inseminated with frozen semen, while they observed no difference in the incidence of uterine fluid in mares inseminated once or more per cycle. The presence of post-insemination uterine fluid is associated with a negative effect on fertility rates and a decrease in conception rates (BARBACINI et al., 2003).

The best time to inseminate a mare with frozen semen is between six hours before or after ovulation (SAMPER & MORRIS, 1998) and, for many years, inseminations were carried out by depositing the semen in the body of the uterus. MORRIS et al. (2000), however, demonstrated pregnancy rates of 64, 75 and 60% in mares inseminated with 1, 5 or 10 million sperm from the same stallion at the utero-tubal junction. It seems that depositing the semen in the uterine horn or close to this junction maximizes the sperm potential, increasing the number of sperm in the oviduct, as well as increasing pregnancy rates in mares inseminated with frozen semen (SAMPER, 2001).

4. NATIVE BREEDS AND THEIR PRESERVATION

In recent years, there has been a growing worldwide concern about the conservation and preservation of native breeds, due to their extinction through absorbent crossbreeding with other breeds. Data from the FAO (2000) show that there are around 40 species of domestic animals (buffalo, goats, horses, oxen, etc.), comprising between 4,500 and 5,000 local breeds and types of animal. Of these breeds, approximately 28% are at risk of extinction, with around half belonging to developing countries. According to REGE & GIBSON (2003), 70% of today's native breeds are found in developing countries.

The conservation of animal genetic resources has become a pressing need due to the great loss of these resources around the world, since their exploitation without criteria and the degradation of the environment imposed by man is widespread in various regions. Different animal genetic resources have not only socio-economic value, but also ethnic and cultural value, including taking part in rituals in some sects and religions (SANTOS et al., 2003).

In Brazil, it can be said that the native breeds that exist today are descendants of animal breeds that were initially brought from Europe by the colonizers, most of which are of Iberian origin. We can mention the Campolina, Mangalarga Marchador, Campeira and Pantaneira breeds as descendants of Spanish horses. However, due to the geoclimatic differences in the breeding regions and the purpose of the breeding by the owners of the animals, breeds emerged that can be called native and which have their own characteristics.

With regard to native breeds, two can be considered vulnerable or threatened with extinction: the Pantaneira breed and the Campeira breed, respectively. Over the years, the Pantaneira breed has developed adaptive characteristics to the Pantanal region's soil and climatic conditions through natural selection (SANTOS et al., 1995) and only failed to become extinct due to the efforts of some breeders and people interested in the breed who mobilized and founded the Brazilian Association of Pantanal Horse Breeders (ABCCP) in 1972. This association currently has approximately 2,600 females and 500 males registered (data provided by ABCCP, 2003).

However, the breeding of the Campeiro horse, which used to be abundant throughout the region of the Catarinense Plateau, the Rio Grande do Sul Plateau and the Campos Gerais do Paranà (Pinhais Region), is currently restricted to the cities of Lages and Curitibanos, both located on the Catarinense Plateau (data provided by the Brazilian Association of Campeiro Horse Breeders - ABRACCCa, 1984). A total of approximately 120 Campeeiro animals were registered in 1985, while in 1998 this number fell to less than 20 animals registered with the association. These figures show that the numbers are worrying and that the breed is heading towards extinction (MC. MANUS et al., 2005).

5. GENERAL OBJECTIVE

To evaluate *in vitro* the effects of reducing the concentration of cryoprotectant after thawing using two commercial diluents on equine semen cryopreserved with diluent containing the cryoprotectant dimethylformamide.

5.1 SPECIFIC OBJECTIVES

To evaluate the sperm parameters of motility and viability after dilution of the cryoprotectant dimethylformamide at 5% to 2.5 and 1.25% concentration in stallions of national breeds using two commercial diluents, as well as to analyze the effect between dilutions and diluents.

6. LITERATURE REVIEW

ABAIGAR, T. et al. Sperm subpopulations in boar (*Sus scrofa*) and gazelle (*gazelle dama mhorr*) semen as revealed by pattern analysis of computer-assisted motility assessments. **Biology Reproduction**. v.60, p. 32-41, 1999.

ABRACCCa, Brazilian Association of Breeders of Champion Horses. Campeiro, the marcher of the Araucarias. **Curitibanos: Pamphlet**, 6p., 1984.

ALVARENGA, M.A. et al. The effect of breed and spermatic parameters over equine semen freezability. In: SYMPOSIUM ON STALLION SEMEN, 1996, Amersfort, **Anais...**; Amersfort, p.82, 1996.

ALVARENGA, M.A., et al. Alternative cryoprotectors for freezing stallion spermatozoa. In: 14th INTERNATIONAL CONGRESS ON ANIMAL REPRODUCTION AND ARTIFICIAL INSEMINATION, 2000. **Proceedings** Stockholm, p.157, 2000.

ALVARENGA, M.A. et al. The use of alternative cryoprotectors for freezing stallion semen. In: Workshop on Transporting Gametes and Embryos, Havemeyer Foundation, 2003. **Proceedings**, p.74-76, 2003.

ALVARENGA, M.A. et al. Amides as cryoprotectants for freezing stallion semen: A review. **An. Reprod. Sci.**, n.89, p.105-113, 2005.

AMANN, R.P.; GRAHAM, J.K. Spermatozoal function. In: McKinnon, AO,Voss JL. **Equine reproduction. Pennsylvania: Lea & Febiger**, chap80, p.715-45, 1993.

AMANN, R.P.; PICKET, B.W. Principles of cryopreservation and a review of cryopreservation of stallion spermatozoa. **J. Equ. Vet. Sci.**, v.7, p.145-173, 1987.

ASHWOOD-SMITH, M.J. Mechanisms of cryoprotectant action. In: BOWLER,K. FULLER, B.J. (Eds.), **Temperature and Animal Cells**. Cambridge, UK, Biologists Ltd. p.395-406, 1987.

AURICH, C. Factors affecting the plasma membrane function of cooled-stored stallion spermatozoa.

Anim. Reprod. Sci., v.89, Issues 1-4, p. 65-75, 2005.

BALL, B.A., VOSS, A. Osmotic tolerance on equine spermatozoa and the effects of soluble cryoprotectants on equine sperm motility, viability and mitochondrial membrane potential. **J. Andrology,** v.22(6), p.1061-9, 2001.

BARBACINI, S. et al. Retrospective study of the incidence of post-insemination uterine fluid in mares with frozen-thawed semen. **J. Equine Vet. Sci.** n.23, p. 493-496, 2003.

BARKER C.A.V., GANDIER, J.C. Pregnancy in a mare resulting from frozen epididymal spermatozoa. **Can J Comp Med Vet Sci,** v.21, p.47-51, 1957.

BLANCHARD, T.L. et al. **Manual of equine reproduction.** Mosby, 2nd ed, 2003.

BOYLE, M.S. Assessing the potential fertility of frozen stallion semen. In: Allen

WR and Wade JF (eds.), **Havemeyer Foundation Monography series** no. 1. R&W

Publications Ltd, Newmarket, p.13-16, 1999.

BRINSKO, S.P., VARNER, D.D. Artificial insemination and preservation of semen. In: BLANCHARD, T.L., VARNER, D.D. Stallion management. **Vet. Clin. North America: Equine Practice**, v.8, n.1, p.205-218, 1992.

BRITO, L.F.C. et al. Comparision of methods to evaluate the plasmalemma of bovine sperm and their relationship with in vitro fertilization rate. **Theriogenology**, v.60, p.1539-1551, 2003.

CHENIER, T. et al. Evaluation of cryoprotective agents for use in the cryopreservation of equine spermatozoa. Proceedings for Annual Meeting, Society for Theriogenology. **Proceedings...**, p.52-53, 1998.

BRAZILIAN COLLEGE OF ANIMAL REPRODUCTION - CBRA. **Manual de exame andrológico e avaliaçâo de sêmen animal**. 2ed.; Belo Horizonte, CBRA, 1998, 49p.

CRISTANELLI, M.J. et al. Fertility of stallion semen processed, frozen and thawed by a new procedure. **Theriogenology**, v.22, p.39-45, 1984.

CROSS, N.L. Role of cholesterol in sperm capacitation, **Biol. Reprod.**, n.59, p. 7-11, 1998.

DE LEEUW, F.E. et al. Cold-induced ultrastructural changes in bull and boar sperm plasma membranes. **Cryobiology,** n.27, p. 171-183, 1990.

DEMICK, D.S. et al. Effect of cooling, storage with glycerolization and spermatozoa number on equine fertility. **J. Anim. Sci.**, v.43, p.633-637, 1976.

DOTT, H.M., FOSTER, G.C. A technique for studying the morphology of mammalian spermatozoa which are eosinophilic in a defferential live and dead stain. **J. Reprod. Fertil.**, v.29, p. 443-446, 1972.

FAO. World watch list for domestic animal diversity. **Edited by B.D. Scherf**, 3rd ed., 744p., Rome, 2000.

FLESCH, F.M., GADELLA, B.M. Dynamics of the mammalian sperm plasma membrane in the process of fertilization, **Biochemica et Biophysica** Acta, n.1469, p.197-235, 2000.

GADELLA, B.M. at el. Capacitation and the acrosome reaction in equine sperm. **Anim. Reprod. Sci.**, v.68, p.249-265, 2001.

GILMORE, J.A. et al. Effects of cryoprotectant solutes on water permeability of human spermatozoa. **Biol. Reprod.**, n.53, p.985-995, 1995.

GIRAUD, M.N. et al. Membrane fluidity predicts the outcome of cryopreservation of human spermatozoa. **Hum. Reprod.**, v.15, p.2160-2164, 2000.

GOMES, G.M. et al. Improvement of stallion spermatozoa preservation with alternative cryoprotectants for Mangalarga Marchador breed. **Theriogenology,** v.58, p.277-9, 2002.

GRAHAM, J.K. Cryopreservation of stallion spermatozoa. **Veterinary Clinical of North American: Equine Practice**, v.12, p.131-147, 1996.

HANADA, A., NAGASE, H. Cryoprotective effects of some amides on rabbit spermatozoa. **J. Reprod. Fert.**, v.60, p.247-252, 1980.

HAARD, M.C.; HAARD, M.G.H. Successful commercialization of frozen stallion semen abroad. **J Reprod Fertil** (Suppl.), n.44, p.647-648, 1991.

HAMMERSTEDT, R.H., GRAHAM, J.K. Cryopreservation of poultry sperm: the enigma of glycerol. **Cryobiology**, n.29, p.26-38, 1992.

HARKEMA, W., BOYLE, M.S. Use of fluorescent stains to assess integrity of equine spermatozoa. **Proc. 12th International Congress on Animal Reproduction**, v.03, p. 1424-1426, 1992.

HARRISON, R.A.P., VICKERS, S.E. Use of fluorescent probes to assess membrane integrity in mammalian spermatozoa. **J. Reprod. Fertil.**, v.88, p.343-352, 1990.

HENRY, M. et al. Post-thaw spermatozoa plasma membrane integrity and motility of stallion semen frozen with different cryoprotectants. **Theriogenology**, n.58, p.245248, 2002.

HOCHACHKA, P.W. Defense strategies against hypoxia and hypothermia. **Science,** v.231, p.234-241, 1986.

HUNTER, R.H.F. Pre ovulatory arrest and periovulatory redistribution of competent spermatozoa in the isthmus of the pig oviduct. **J. Reprod. Fertil.**, n.72, pgs. 203211, 1984.

JASKO, D.J. et al. Pregnancy rates utilizing fresh, cooled and frozen-thawed stallion semen.In: 38th Ann. Conv. AAEP. **Proceedings,** p.649-660, 1992.

JEYENDRAN, R.S., GRAHAM, E.F. An evaluation of cryoprotective compounds on bovine spermatozoa . **Cryobiology,** v. 17, p.458-464, 1980.

KATILA, T. Neutrophils in uterine fluid after insemination with fresh live spermatozoa or with killed spermatozoa. **Pferdeheilkunde**, n. 13, p.54, 1997.

KEITH, S.L. **Evaluation of new cryoprotectants for the preservation of equine semen**. 1998, Master Thesis, Colorado State University, Colorado.

KOTILAINEN, T. et al. Sperm-induced leukocytosis in the equine uterus. **Theriogenology**, n.41, p.629-636, 1994.

LOOMIS, P.R. The equine frozen semen industry. **Anim. Reprod. Sci.**, v.68, p.191-200, 2001.

LOOMIS, P.R, SQUIRES, E.L. Frozen semen management in equine breeding programs. Captured on June 25, 2005. Available on the Internet. http://www.joumals.elsevierhealth.com/periodicals/the.

MARTIN, C.E.G. et al. Viability of equine spermatozoa cryopreserved in diluent containing Low Density Iipoprotein. In: Congr. Bras. de Reprod. Animal. **Anais...,** v.16, p.227, Goiânia, GO, 2005. (Abstracts)

MARTIN, J.C. et al. Centrifugation of stallion semen and its storage in large volume straw. **J. Reprod. Fertil. Suppl.,** n.27, p.47-51, 1979.

MC. MANUS et al. Morphological characterization of Campeiro breed horses. **Ver. Bras. Zootec.**, v.34, n.5. p.1553-1562, 2005.

MEDEIROS, A.S.L. et al. Cryopreservation of stallion sperm using different amides. **Theriogenology**, n.58, p.273-276, 2002.

MEDEIROS, A.S.L. et al. Evaluation of the acrosomal integrity of spermatozoa from sires cryopreserved with cryoprotectants based on amides and glycerol. **Rev. Bras. Reprod. Anim.**, v.27, n.3, p. 353-354, 2003.

MELLO, F.G. et al. Effects of the fractional addition of dimethylformamide to the diluting medium and two cooling curves on the preservation of the viability of frozen equine spermatozoa. In: Congr. Bras. de Reprod. Animal. **Anais,** v.16, p.268, Goiânia, GO, 2005. (Abstracts)

MELO,C.M. et al. Effect of different centrifugation diluents and cryoprotectants on the freezing of equine semen. In: Congr. Bras. de Reprod. Animal. **Anais.,** v.16, p.185, Goiânia, GO, 2005. (Abstracts)

METCALF, E.L. The effect of post-insemination endometritis on fertility of frozen stallion semen. In: 46th Ann. Conv. AAEP. **Proceedings.** p.332-400, 2000.

MINELLI, A. et al. Occurrence of prostasome-like membrane vesicles in equine seminal plasma. **J**

Reprod Fertil, v.2, n.114, p.237-243, 1998.

MOFFET, P.D. et al. Comparision of dimethyl-formamide and glycerol for cryopreservation of equine spermatozoa. Proc. Soc. For Theriogenology Ann. Conf. **Abstract...,** p.42, 2003.

MORRIS, L.H.A. et al. Hysteroscopic insemonation of small numbers of spermatozoa at the uterotubal junction of preovulatory mares. **J. Reprod. Fertil.** , v. 118, p.95-100, 2000.

NEILD, D.M., et al. The HOS test and its relationship to fertility in the stallion. **Andrologia,** n.32, p.351-355, 1999.

NEVES NETO, J.R. et al. Structural and functional evaluation of the equine sperm cell against different cryoprotective substances. Brazilian Society of Embryo Transfer. **Acta Scientia Veterinariae,**. n. 32 (Supl.), p.175, 2004.

OLIVEIRA, J.V. et al. Effect of cryoprotectant on donkey semen freezability and fertility. **Anim. Reprod. Sci.** n. 94, p. 82-84, 2006.

PICKETT, B.W., AMANN, R.P. Cryopreservation of semen. In: MCKINNON, A.O., VOSS, J.L. **Equine Reproduction**, Philadelphia: Lea & Febiger (ed.), p.769-789, 1993.

PICKETT, B.W. Pregnancy rates utilizing fresh, cooled and frozen-thawed stallion semen. In: 38th Ann. Conv. AAEP. **Proceedings.** p.649-660, 1992.

PICKETT, B.W. Principles of cryopreservation**.** In: TECHNIQUES FOR FREEZING MAMMALIAN EMBRYOS. **Proceedings...,** Fort Collins: Colorado State University, p.1-5, 1998.

REGE, J.E.O., GIBSON, J.P. Animal genetic resources and economic development: issues in relation to economic valuation. **Ecological Economics**, v.45, p.319-330, 2003.

SAMPER, J.C., MORRIS, C.A. Current methodology for stallion semen cryopreservation: an international survey. **Theriogenology**, v.49, p. 895-904, 1998.

SAMPER, J.C. Management and fertility of mares bred with frozen semen. **Anim. Reprod., Sci.,** v.68, p. 219-228, 2001.

SANTOS, S.A. et al. Evaluation and conservation of the Pantanal horse. **Corumbà: EMBRAPA-CPAC**, technical circular n.21, 40p., 1995.

SANTOS, S.A. et al. Estratégias de Conservaçao *in situ* do Cavalo Pantaneiro. **Corumbà:EMBRAPA Pantanal**, ISSN 1517-1973, n.55, 30p., 2003.

SCHÀFER-SOMI, S., AURICH, C. Use of a new computer-assisted sperm analyzer for the assessment of motility and viability of dog spermatozoa and evaluation of four different semen extenders for predilution. **Anim. Reprod. Sci.**, doi: 10.1016/janireprosci.2005.03.019, 2006.

SILVA, J.A.B. et al. Cryopreservation of equine semen using different cryoprotectants. Master's thesis - FAV-UNB Postgraduate Course, Brasilia, DF, 2005.

SNOECK, P.P.N. et al. Effect of three thawing temperatures on equine spermatozoa frozen with different cryoprotective agents. **Rev. Bras. Reprod. Anim.,** v.26, n.3, p.454-5, 2002

SQUIRES, E.L. et al. Cooled and frozen Stallion Semen. **Fort Collins: Animal Reproduction and Biotechnology Laboratory**, 1999. (Handout).

SQUIRES, E.L. Integration of future biotechnologies into the equine industry. **Ani. Reprod. Sci.,** v. 89, Issues 1-4, p.187-198, oct.2005.

STRYER, L. **Introduction to the study of biological membranes.** In: . Biochemistry. 3.ed. Rio de Janeiro: Guanabara Koogan, ch. 12, p. 230-56, 1992.

THOMASSEN, R. Insemination with stallion semen frozen in 0.5 ml straws. **Reprod. Dom. Anim.** v.28, p.289-293, 1993.

THURSTON, L.M., et al., Sources of variation in the morphological characteristics of sperm subpopulations assessed objectively by a novel automated sperm morphology analysis system. **J. Rerpod. Fert.,** n.117, p. 271-280, 1999.

TORRES-BOGGINO, F., et al. Relationship among seminal characteristics, fertility and suitability for semen preservation in draft stallions. **J. Vet. Med. Sci.,** n.57, p.225229, 1994.

TROEDSSON, M.H.T. et al. Mechanism of sperm-induced endometritis in the mare. **Biol. Reprod. Suppl.**, v.52, p.307, 1995.

VERSTEGEN, J. et al. Computer assisted semen analyzers in andrology research and veterinary practice. **Theriogenology,** n.57, v.1, p.149-179, 2002.

VIDAMENT, M.et al. Motility and fertility of stallion semen frozen with glycerol and/or dimetyl formamide. **Theriogenology**, n.58, p.1-3, 2002.

VIZCARRA, J.A., FORD,J.J. Validation of the sperm mobility assay in boars and stallions. **Theriogenology,** n.66, p.1091-1097, 2006.

WATSON, P.F. The effects of cold shock on sperm cell membranes. In: MORRIS, G.J.

& CLARKE, A. **Effects of low temperature on biological membranes.** Academic Press, New York, p.189-218, 1981.

WATSON, P.F. Recent developments and concepts in the cryopreservation of spermatozoa and the assesment of their post-thawing function. **Reprod. Fert. Dev.,** v.7, p.871-891, 1995.

WATSON, P.F. The causes of reduced fertility with cryopreserved semen. **An. Reprod. Sci**. n.60-61, pgs.481-492, 2000.

WILMUT I., POLGE, C. The low temperatures preservation of boar spermatozoa frozen and thawed in the presence of permeating agents. **Cryobiology,** v.14, p.471-8, 1977.

YANAGUIMACHI, R. In. E. KNOBIL, J.D. NEILL (Eds.), **The Physiology of Reproduction**, Raven Press, New York, p.189-317, 1994.

ZÙCCARI, C.E.S.N. **Effect of cryopreservation on the structural integrity of the equine sperm cell.** Thesis (PhD) - Postgraduate Course in Animal Reproduction, FMVZ - UNESP, Botucatu, SP, 1998.

7. SINGLE CHAPTER

Effect of dilution of the cryoprotectant dimethylformamide on equine semen samples thawed using two different commercial diluents

Dilution effect of dimethylformamyde cryoprotectant from post thawed equine semen samples using two different commercial diluents

Marina Ferreira Zimmermann; Adalberto Farinasso, Cely Marini Melo, Frederico Ozanam Papa, Jairo Pereira Neves

Paper submitted to the Ciência Rural journal of the University of Santa Maria, RS.

SUMMARY

The aim of this study was to evaluate motility parameters and in vitro *viability when diluting the 5% post-thaw cryoprotectant dimethylformamide to concentrations of 2.5 and 1.25%, using two commercial diluents added to cryopreserved equine semen. After thawing, the samples were diluted in order to maintain the final concentrations (2.5 and 1.25%) of cryoprotectant, using two commercial diluents (FR4® and Botu-Crio®) at two times: initial (Ti) and final (Tf). Thirteen different ejaculate samples from five national breed sires were used. Motility parameters were observed using computerized analysis and plasma membrane integrity using epifluorescence microscopy. There was an improvement in total and progressive sperm motility parameters at the final time (P<0.05) with Botu-Crio® diluent compared to FR4®. There was no difference, P>0.05, between the treatments in terms of plasma membrane integrity.*

Keywords: *equine, diluent, cryoprotectant, freezing. thawing.*

INTRODUCTION

The number of mares inseminated with frozen semen is increasing and this is stimulating and attracting greater investment in the field of equine reproduction (SQUIRES,

2005). Semen freezing promotes greater exchange between stud farms in different regions and countries, selects individuals for fertility and freezability, and also helps conserve endangered species (WATSON, 2000).

There is individual variability in semen freezability due to genetic and environmental factors. In the equine species, a large number of stallions have post-thaw semen characteristics, such as motility and membrane integrity, which are unsuitable for use (SQUIRES et al., 1999). There are cases where post-insemination uterine inflammation, acute endometritis, appears to be more long-lasting depending on the cryoprotective agent used and the number of sperm inseminated with frozen semen (METCALF, 2000).

Most studies aimed at increasing the survival of frozen and thawed spermatozoa seek to minimize oxidative stress and reduce osmotic stress (SQUIRES, 2005). Semen collection, the addition of diluents, centrifugation, refrigeration, freezing and thawing cause damage to the plasma membrane of spermatozoa (AURICH, 2005).

Equine spermatozoa seem to withstand a range between 150-900 mOsm and when the cell volume exceeds the lithium volume of the cell, rupture of the plasma membrane occurs, resulting in loss of viability (POMMER et al., 2002). DE LEEUW et al. (1990) suggest that changes in the phospholipid layer caused by phase-separation events during the cryopreservation process affect osmotic properties. Especially for equine spermatozoa, whose membrane permeability is affected by the cold shock induced by rapid freezing at temperatures close to zero (DEVIREDDY et al., 2002).

According to ALVARENGA et al. (2005), the lower viscosity and lower molecular weight of amides favor greater permeability of these components within the plasma membrane. BALL & VO (2001) reported that rapid removal of cryoprotectants results in a relative hyposmotic shock on dilution in isotonic extender media or in the fluids of the mare's uterine tract. This is reflected in the rapid loss of sperm motility, membrane integrity and mitochondrial membrane potential (POMMER et al., 2002).

The aim of this study was to evaluate *in vitro* the effects of reducing the concentration of the cryoprotectant dimethylformamide at 5% post-thaw to 2.5 and 1.25% using two commercial diluents on cryopreserved equine semen.

MATERIAL AND METHODS

Five stallions of national breeds were used: Pantaneira (2), Campeira (2) and Campolina (1), aged between 4 and 15 years, suitable for reproduction and with good fertility. Freezing was carried out at the Animal Reproduction Laboratory of Embrapa Recursos Genéticos e Biotecnologia / CENARGEN, Fazenda Experimental Sucupira, Brasilia - DF.

The samples were collected using a Botucatu model artificial vagina and a nylon filter to remove the gel fraction. After collection, the following characteristics were examined: volume, appearance, color, motility (0-100), vigor (05) and sperm concentration (1:20) using a microscope with a 20X objective.

The semen was diluted with skimmed milk-based extender (1:1 ratio) and centrifuged at 600g/10 min. The supernatant was removed and the *pellets* resuspended in FR4 freezing medium® (Nutricell, Campinas/SP) containing 5% dimethyl-formamide cryoprotectant (SIGMA-ALDRICHT®). Packaging was carried out in 0.5mL straws identified and sealed with polyvinyl alcohol and with a final concentration of 100×10^6 sperm/mL. The straws were cooled at 5°C for 60 min. in a domestic refrigerator, then frozen in liquid nitrogen vapor (distributed in a Styrofoam box) and placed on a support at a height of 5cm above the liquid level of N_2 and a temperature close to -120°C, for 20 min. After this time, the straws were immersed in liquid nitrogen at a temperature close to - 196°C and stored in a cryobiological tank.

The semen samples were analyzed at the Andrology Laboratory of the Department of Radiology and Animal Reproduction of the Faculty of Veterinary Medicine and Zootechny - UNESP / Campus Botucatu. Thirteen samples from 13 different ejaculates were thawed. The straws were thawed at a temperature of 45°C for 20 seconds and the semen was stored in microcentrifuge tubes previously heated to 37°C and separated into five aliquots, as follows:

C = control (semen); **1) FR50** = 50μL of semen + 50μL of FR4® diluent / 50% dilution; **2) BOT50** = 50μL of semen + 50μL of Botu-Crio® diluent / 50% dilution; **3) FR25** = FR 50 + 100μL of FR4® diluent / 25% dilution; **4) BOT25** = BOT 25 + 100μL of Botu-Crio® diluent / 25% dilution.

*Both diluters, FR4® (Nutricell) and Botu-Crio® (Biotech-Botucatu-Ltda/ME, Brazil) contained no cryoprotectant.

The initial analyses were carried out 10 min after the dilutions (stabilization time) on the samples, which were then placed in a dry water bath at 37°C. Evaluations were carried out using computerized motility analysis (CASA).

The samples were analyzed according to the following parameters: total motility (MT%), progressive motility (MP%), average velocity (VAPμm/s), progressive velocity (VSLμm/s), curvilinear velocity (VCLμm/s), lateral head displacement (ALHμm), flagellar beat frequency (BCF Hz), amount of rapid spermatozoa (RAP%), at times Ti (initial) and Tf (final, 1h after dilutions).

To assess the integrity of the plasma membrane (IMP), the staining technique described by ZÙCCARI (1998) was used: carboxyfluorescein solution (20μL), propidium iodide solution (10μL), formaldehyde solution (10μL) and sodium citrate solution (0.96mL). 40μL of each treatment was added to the solution described and then evaluated under epifluorescence microscopy, analyzing 200 cells/treatment/slide. Spermatozoa stained green were considered to have an integral membrane and those stained red had a damaged membrane.

Tukey's test was used for statistical analysis to compare the means of the motility and plasma membrane integrity variables. The Dunnet test was used to compare each of the four treatments with the control and analysis of variance was used to compare the effects between diluents and between dilutions. All at the initial (Ti) and final (Tf) time points.

The SPSS 13.0 program (Statistical Program for Social Sciences) was used for the statistical analysis, considering a significance level of 5%.

RESULTS AND DISCUSSION

This study evaluated sperm motility and viability parameters after thawing and diluting the semen, keeping the final cryoprotectant concentrations at 2.5 and 1.25%, using the diluents FR4® and Botu-Crio®. There was no effect of sire and/or between ejaculates from the same sire. The average total sperm motility (TM) and progressive sperm motility (PM) in the control animals studied were 59% and 16%, respectively, and 48% plasma membrane integrity in the epifluorescence test (IMP).

There was a significant difference between the means of the treatments (control, 1, 2, 3 and 4) for MP, VSL, ALH and BCF in the initial time (Ti), with no significant difference (P>0.05) for MT, VAP, VCL, RAP and IMP. At the end time (Tf), significant differences (P<0.05) were observed for MT, MP, VAP, VSL, VCL, BCF and RAP; no significant difference (P>0.05) was observed for IMP, between the averages of the treatments (Figure 1; Table 2).

There was a difference (P<0.05) in MP when using Botu-Crio diluent® : control (15.8%), BOT50 (28.5%) and BOT25 (25.9%) and ALH (7.7; 6.6; 6.9, respectively). There was also a difference in BCF between the control and BOT50, FR25 and BOT25; and in VSL between the control and all the treatments. There was no difference (P>0.05) in MT, VAP, VCL and RAP (Figure 1; Table 2). In the membrane integrity test (IMP), there was no difference between treatments. The results differ from those observed by WESSEL & BALL (2004) in which the rapid removal of glycerol from fresh equine semen resulted in a reduction in sperm motility and membrane integrity, while the serial dilution of glycerol from the same semen resulted in an improvement in the maintenance of both sperm motility and membrane integrity, concluding that there was no similar beneficial effect when serial dilution was carried out with cryopreserved semen.

For the final time (Tf), there was a difference (P<0.05) in MP between control, FR50, BOT50, FR25 and BOT25, also for VAP, VSL, VCL and RAP; in MT between control and FR50, BOT50 and BOT25; for BCF between control and BOT50 and BOT25. There was no difference (P>0.05) for IMP and ALH (Figure 1; Table 2).

When comparing diluents and dilutions in a factorial (4X4), there was a difference (P<0.05) only for ALH and BCF in the initial time (Ti) between the diluents tested, with no difference (P>0.05) between dilutions. At the end time (Tf), for the averages between diluents, there was a difference (P<0.05) in MT (37% and 42%), MP (12% and 17%), ALH (7.5 and 7.0) and BCF (25 and 29), respectively, with FR4® and Botu-Crio® ; there was no difference (P>0.05) in VAP, VSL, VCL, RAP and IMP. There was no difference between dilutions (50% or 25%) for all the parameters analyzed, data which agrees with that of WESSEL & BALL (2004) in which the type of dilution in their experiment after thawing did not affect the total and progressive sperm motility of the spermatozoa, although they did observe an effect between sires. In the present study, there was no interaction between diluents and dilutions at either time (Table 1).

The analysis carried out at the final time, Ihora after the first evaluations, indicated an improvement and difference (P<0.05) in all the parameters analyzed, except lateral head displacement (ALH) and membrane integrity (IMP), indicating that a dilution of the cryoprotectant after thawing can increase the survival of sperm cells without damaging their membranes. There was also an improvement (P<0.05) in MP and MT parameters for semen treated with Botu-Crio diluent® when compared to FR4®. A study by MELO et al. (2006) using the Botu-Crio® diluent showed that, although the amides used in their experiment had similar chemical structures, a combination of this diluent and 4% dimethylacetamide showed superior sperm protection during the freezing process compared to the combination of the diluent and 4% dimethylformamide, although there was no significant difference in the fertility test between the two.

Some studies have reported the theoretical benefits of serial dilution to remove cryoprotectants from frozen semen in humans, but there are few experimental results on the effects on sperm cells, making the data still not very consistent (GAO et al., 1995; GILMORE et al., 1997). GAO et al. (1995) observed that sperm motility is much more sensitive to anisosmotic conditions than membrane integrity; sperm motility has been shown to be even more sensitive to hypo- than hypertonic conditions in human cells. According to BALL & VO (2001), rapid removal of permeable cryoprotectants results in possible hyposmotic shock when diluted in extension media or in the fluids of the mares' reproductive tract.

CONCLUSIONS

Post-thawing dilutions of equine semen cryopreserved with 5% dimethylformamide cryoprotectant using two commercial diluents (Botu-Crio® and FR4®) provided greater sperm cell survival. The diluent Botu-Crio® provided better results than the diluent FR4® . These results should be confirmed *in in vivo* tests.

ACKNOWLEDGMENTS

To CNPq for the financial support and scholarships.

REFERENCES

ALVARENGA, M.A. et al. Amides as cryoprotectants for freezing stallion semen: A review. **Animal Reproduction Science**, n.89, p.105-113, 2005.

AURICH, C. Factors affecting the plasma membrane function of cooled-stored stallion spermatozoa. **Animimal Reproduction Science**, v.89, Issues 1-4, p. 65-75, 2005.

BALL, B.A.; VO, A. Osmotic tolerance of equine spermatozoa and the effects of soluble cryoprotectants on equine sperm motility, viability, and mithocondrial membrane potential. **Journal of Andrology**, n.22, p. 1061-1069, 2001.

DE LEEUW, F.E. et al. Cold-induced ultrastructural changes in bull and boar sperm plasma membranes. **Cryobiology,** n.27, p. 171-183, 1990.

DEVIREDDY, R.V. et al. Cryopreservation of equine sperm: optimal cooling rates in the presence and absence of cryoprotective agents determined using differential scanning calorimetry. **Biology Reproduction**, n.66, p.222-231, 2002.

GAO, D.Y. et al. Prevention of osmotic injury to human spermatozoa during addition and removal of glycerol. **Human Reproduction**, n.10, p.1109-1122, 1995. (Abstract)

GILMORE, J.A. et al. Determination of optimal cryoprotectants and procedures for their addition and removal from human spermatozoa. **Human Reproduction**, n.12, p.112118, 1997.

MELO, C.M. et al. Use of different centrifugation diluents and cryoprotectants on the fertility of frozen equine semen. **Acta Scientiae Veterinariae**, 34 (supl.1), p.566, 2006.

METCALF, E.L. The effect of post-insemination endometritis on fertility of frozen stallion semen. In: 46th Ann. Conv. AAEP. **Proceedings,** p.332-400, 2000.

POMMER, A.C. et al. The role of osmotic resistance on equine spermatozoal function. **Theriogenology**, n.58, p. 1373-1384, 2002.

SQUIRES, E.L. Integration of future biotechnologies into the equine industry. **Animal Reproduction Science**, v. 89, Issues 1-4, p.187-198, oct.2005.

SPSS 13.0, Statistical Program for Social Sciences for windows.

WATSON, P.F. The causes of reduced fertility with cryopreserved semen. **Animal Reproduction Science**, n.60-61, pgs.481-492, 2000.

WESSEL, M.T.; BALL, B.A. Step-wise dilution for removal of glycerol from fresh and cryopreserved equine spermatozoa. **Animal Reproduction Science**, n.84, p.147-156, 2004.

ZÙCCARI, C.E.S.N. **Effect of cryopreservation on the structural integrity of the equine sperm cell.** Thesis (PhD) - Postgraduate Course in Animal Reproduction, FMVZ - UNESP, Botucatu, SP, 1998.

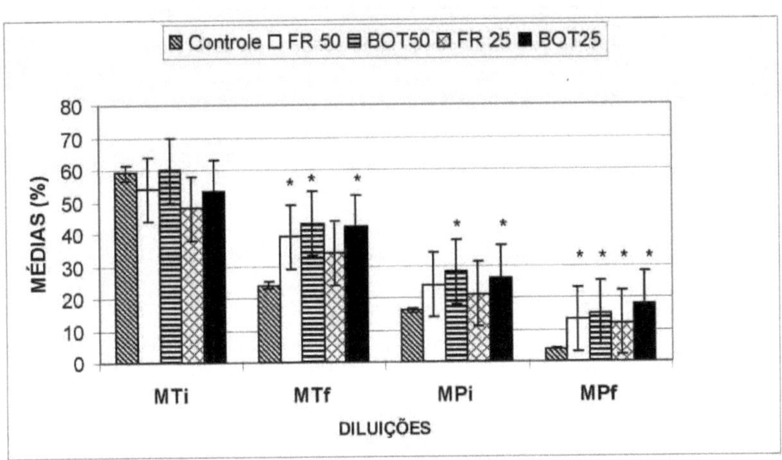

Figure 1: Graphical expression of the means in percentages, using Dunnett's test, comparing the control with the other treatments and using the variables MTi: initial total motility, MTf: final total motility, MPi: initial progressive motility, MPf: final progressive motility; * Represents statistical difference ($P < 0.05$).

Table 1: Comparison of means (±) between diluents and dilutions of total and progressive sperm motility and plasma membrane integrity of equine semen de- iced and treated with different diluents (FR4® and BOTUCRIO®) and dilutions (50 and 25%) at the final time (Tf):

	FR50	FR25	TOTAL FR	BOT50	BOT25	TOTAL BOT	TOTAL50	TOTAL25	TOTAL %
MT	39,0	34,5	37,2	43,1	41,8	42,4*	41,2	39,2	40,2
MP	13,2	11,7	12,6	14,9	18,5	16,8*	14,1	16,1	15,0
IMP	40,2	37,8	39,3	42,9	40,3	41,5	41,6	39,4	40,6

MT: total motility; MP: progressive motility; IMP: membrane integrity

values with significant difference ($P < 0.05$)

Table 2: Means (±), standard deviation and significant difference (P<0.05) of the treatments of thawed and treated equine semen, evaluated by CASA and the epifluorescence test (IMP) at the initial (Ti) and final (Tf) times:

T			INITIAL	(T=0)		T FINAL		(T=1)		
Var. indep.	Control	FR 50	BOT50	FR 25	BOT25	Control	FR 50	BOT50	FR 25	BOT 25
MT (%)	$59 \pm 8,8^a$	$53 \pm 8,5^a$	$60 \pm 9,1^a$	$48 \pm 6,9^a$	$53 \pm 12,5^a$	$24 \pm 9,3^a$	$39 \pm 7,7^b$	$43 \pm 9,18^b$	$34 \pm 10,2^{a,b}$	$41 \pm 4,6^b$
MP (%)	$16 \pm 4,6^a$	$24 \pm 3,9^{a,b}$	$28 \pm 7,5^b$	$21 \pm 6,8^{a,b}$	$26 \pm 9,2^b$	$4 \pm 5,5^a$	$13 \pm 4,8^{b,c}$	$15 \pm 5,8^{b,c}$	$11 \pm 4,58^b$	$18 \pm 3,8^c$
VAP (µm/s)	$97 \pm 10,5^a$	$106 \pm 7,7^a$	$103 \pm 5,4^a$	$104 \pm 10,3^a$	$101 \pm 11,6^a$	$67 \pm 7,1^a$	$91 \pm 10,2^b$	$89 \pm 8,4^b$	$94 \pm 5,52^b$	$95 \pm 6,6^b$
VSL (µm/s)	$69 \pm 7,6^a$	$81 \pm 4,2^b$	$80 \pm 5,6^b$	$81 \pm 9,0^b$	$79 \pm 9,6^b$	$47 \pm 5,6^a$	$69 \pm 8,3^b$	$68 \pm 7,34^b$	$71 \pm 5,01^b$	$74 \pm 5,8^b$
LCV (µm/s)	$180 \pm 18,8^a$	$197 \pm 12,4^a$	$181 \pm 12,8^a$	$171 \pm 65,6^a$	$176 \pm 22,6^a$	$133 \pm 14,3^a$	$169 \pm 21,3^b$	$168 \pm 18,2^b$	$175 \pm 10,3^b$	$169 \pm 15,2^b$
ALH (µm/s)	$7,7 \pm 0,2^{b,c}$	$8,1 \pm 0,4^c$	$6,7 \pm 0,5^a$	$8,0 \pm 0,9^c$	$6,9 \pm 0,9^{a,b}$	$7,3 \pm 0,4^a$	$7,3 \pm 0,6^a$	$7,3 \pm 0,7^a$	$7,7 \pm 0,57^a$	$6,8 \pm 0,7^a$
BCF	$24 \pm 3,1^a$	$26 \pm 2,0^a$	$30 \pm 2,8^b$	$27 \pm 1,6^{a,b}$	$30 \pm 3,6^b$	$21 \pm 5,7^a$	$26 \pm 3,3^b$	$28 \pm 4,4^b$	$23 \pm 2,51^{a,b}$	$29 \pm 4,3^b$
APR (%)	$41 \pm 9,9^a$	$42 \pm 7,4^a$	$49 \pm 8,4^a$	$39 \pm 6,2^a$	$41 \pm 12,5^a$	$10 \pm 5,4^a$	$28 \pm 8,7^b$	$29 \pm 8,6^b$	$24 \pm 7,88^b$	$31 \pm 3,5^b$
IMP (%)	$48 \pm 6,9^a$	$49 \pm 8,2^a$	$50 \pm 6,2^a$	$46 \pm 5,7^a$	$46 \pm 7,9^a$	$36 \pm 12,7^a$	$40 \pm 6,3^a$	$43 \pm 3,8^a$	$38 \pm 7,34^a$	$40 \pm 7,0^a$

MT: initial total motility; MP: progressive motility; VAP: average velocity; VSL: progressive velocity; VCL: curvilinear velocity;

ALH: lateral head displacement; BCF: flagellar beat frequency; RAP: number of fast spermatozoa; IMP: membrane integrity; Values with different letters (a, b, c) on the same line are statistically different (P<0.05).

ANNEXES:

Annex I:

ADJUSTMENT OF HTMA-IVOS-10 FOR SEMINAL ANALYSIS IN HORSES

Contrast of the cells in relation to the field	60 pixels
Minimum cell size	3 pixels
Contact for real estate cells	30 pixels
Lower limit for rectilinear index	80%
Reference for average speed (VAP)	<70 µm/s
High speed reference (VCL)	<30 µm/s
Slow speed reference (VSL)	<20 µm/s
Lower size limit	0,62 pixels
Upper size limit	2,98 pixels
Lower intensity limit	0,24
Upper intensity limit	1,19
Lower stretch limit	0%
Upper stretch limit	100%
Slow counted as mobile	No
Magnification	1,95

PREPARATION OF FLUORESCENT PROBES

SOLUTIONS	CONSTITUENTS	QUANTITY
IP stock	Propidium Iodide[1]	10mg
	Physiological Solution	20mL
CFDA stock	Diacetate Carboxyfluorescein[2]	9.2mg
	DMSO	20mL
Formaldehyde stock	Formalin 40%	1mL
	Physiological Solution	79mL
Sodium Citrate stock	Sodium Citrate	3g
	Physiological Solution	100mL

[1] P 4170 - Sigma [2] C 5041 - Sigma

WORK SOLUTION

SOLUTION	QUANTITY
3% Sodium Citrate Solution	0.96mL
Formaldehyde solution	10 µl
Propidium Iodide Solution	10 µl
Solving Carboxyfluorescein	20 µl

More Books!

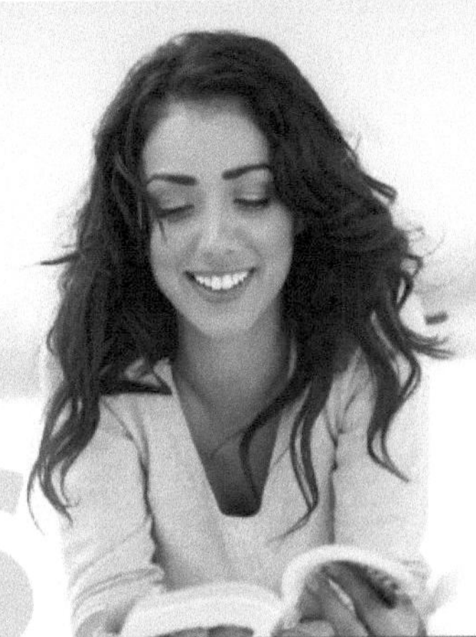

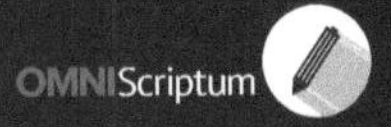

info@omniscriptum.com
www.omniscriptum.com
OMNIScriptum

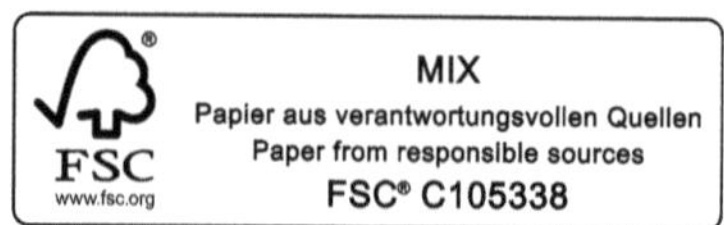

Printed by Books on Demand GmbH, Norderstedt / Germany